THIS BOOK
BELONGS TO

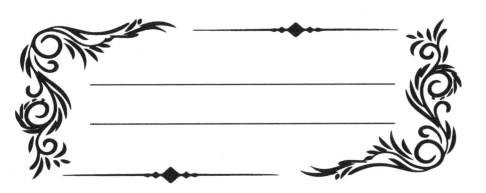

WEIGHT LOSS
♡ Tracker ♡

DATE	-/+	WEIGHT	NOTES

WEIGHT LOSS
♡ Tracker ♡

DATE	-/+	WEIGHT	NOTES

WEIGHT LOSS
♡ Tracker ♡

DATE			-/+		WEIGHT	NOTES

WEIGHT LOSS
♡ Tracker ♡

DATE			-/+		WEIGHT	NOTES

WEIGHT LOSS
♡ Tracker ♡

DATE			-/+		WEIGHT	NOTES

WEIGHT LOSS
♡ Tracker ♡

DATE	-/+	WEIGHT	NOTES

WEIGHT LOSS
♡ Tracker ♡

DATE	-/+	WEIGHT	NOTES

WEIGHT LOSS
♡ Tracker ♡

DATE	-/+		WEIGHT	NOTES

WEIGHT LOSS
Tracker

DATE	-/+	WEIGHT	NOTES

WEIGHT LOSS
Tracker

DATE	-/+	WEIGHT	NOTES

WEIGHT LOSS
♡ Tracker ♡

DATE			-/+		WEIGHT	NOTES

WEIGHT LOSS
♡ Tracker ♡

DATE			-/+		WEIGHT	NOTES

WEIGHT LOSS
♡ Tracker ♡

DATE			-/+		WEIGHT	NOTES

WEIGHT LOSS
♡ Tracker ♡

DATE	-/+	WEIGHT	NOTES

WEIGHT LOSS
Tracker

DATE	-/+	WEIGHT	NOTES

WEIGHT LOSS
♡ Tracker ♡

DATE			-/+		WEIGHT	NOTES

WEIGHT LOSS
♡ Tracker ♡

DATE	-/+	WEIGHT	NOTES

WEIGHT LOSS
Tracker

DATE	-/+		WEIGHT	NOTES

WEIGHT LOSS
♡ Tracker ♡

DATE	-/+	WEIGHT	NOTES

WEIGHT LOSS
♡ Tracker ♡

DATE	-/+	WEIGHT	NOTES

WEIGHT LOSS
♡ Tracker ♡

DATE			-/+		WEIGHT	NOTES

WEIGHT LOSS
♡ Tracker ♡

DATE	-/+	WEIGHT	NOTES

WEIGHT LOSS
♡ Tracker ♡

DATE			-/+	WEIGHT	NOTES

WEIGHT LOSS
♡ Tracker ♡

DATE	-/+	WEIGHT	NOTES

WEIGHT LOSS
♡ Tracker ♡

DATE	-/+	WEIGHT	NOTES

WEIGHT LOSS
♡ Tracker ♡

DATE	-/+	WEIGHT	NOTES

WEIGHT LOSS
♡ Tracker ♡

DATE			-/+		WEIGHT	NOTES

WEIGHT LOSS
♡ Tracker ♡

DATE	-/+	WEIGHT	NOTES

WEIGHT LOSS
♡ Tracker ♡

DATE	-/+	WEIGHT	NOTES

WEIGHT LOSS
♡ Tracker ♡

DATE	-/+	WEIGHT	NOTES

WEIGHT LOSS
♡ Tracker ♡

DATE	-/+	WEIGHT	NOTES

WEIGHT LOSS
♡ Tracker ♡

DATE			-/+		WEIGHT	NOTES

WEIGHT LOSS
♡ Tracker ♡

DATE	-/+	WEIGHT	NOTES

WEIGHT LOSS
♡ Tracker ♡

DATE			-/+		WEIGHT	NOTES

WEIGHT LOSS
♡ Tracker ♡

DATE			-/+	WEIGHT	NOTES

WEIGHT LOSS
Tracker

DATE	-/+	WEIGHT	NOTES

WEIGHT LOSS
♡ Tracker ♡

DATE	-/+	WEIGHT	NOTES

WEIGHT LOSS
♡ Tracker ♡

DATE	-/+	WEIGHT	NOTES

WEIGHT LOSS
♡ Tracker ♡

DATE	-/+	WEIGHT	NOTES

WEIGHT LOSS
♡ Tracker ♡

DATE	-/+	WEIGHT	NOTES

WEIGHT LOSS
♡ Tracker ♡

DATE			-/+	WEIGHT	NOTES

WEIGHT LOSS
Tracker

DATE	-/+	WEIGHT	NOTES

WEIGHT LOSS
♡ Tracker ♡

DATE	-/+	WEIGHT	NOTES

WEIGHT LOSS
Tracker

DATE	-/+	WEIGHT	NOTES

WEIGHT LOSS
♡ Tracker ♡

DATE			-/+		WEIGHT	NOTES

WEIGHT LOSS
♡ Tracker ♡

DATE			-/+	WEIGHT	NOTES

WEIGHT LOSS
♡ Tracker ♡

DATE	-/+	WEIGHT	NOTES

WEIGHT LOSS
♡ Tracker ♡

DATE	-/+	WEIGHT	NOTES

WEIGHT LOSS
♡ Tracker ♡

DATE			-/+		WEIGHT	NOTES

WEIGHT LOSS
♡ Tracker ♡

DATE	-/+	WEIGHT	NOTES

WEIGHT LOSS
♡ Tracker ♡

DATE	-/+	WEIGHT	NOTES

WEIGHT LOSS
♡ Tracker ♡

DATE	-/+	WEIGHT	NOTES

WEIGHT LOSS
♡ Tracker ♡

DATE	-/+	WEIGHT	NOTES

WEIGHT LOSS
♡ Tracker ♡

DATE			-/+		WEIGHT	NOTES

WEIGHT LOSS
♡ Tracker ♡

DATE	-/+	WEIGHT	NOTES

WEIGHT LOSS
Tracker

DATE			-/+		WEIGHT	NOTES

WEIGHT LOSS
♡ Tracker ♡

DATE			-/+		WEIGHT	NOTES

WEIGHT LOSS
♡ Tracker ♡

DATE			-/+		WEIGHT	NOTES

WEIGHT LOSS
♡ Tracker ♡

DATE	-/+	WEIGHT	NOTES

WEIGHT LOSS
Tracker

DATE	-/+	WEIGHT	NOTES

WEIGHT LOSS
Tracker

DATE	-/+	WEIGHT	NOTES

WEIGHT LOSS
♡ Tracker ♡

DATE	-/+	WEIGHT	NOTES

WEIGHT LOSS
♡ Tracker ♡

DATE	-/+	WEIGHT	NOTES

WEIGHT LOSS
♡ Tracker ♡

DATE	-/+	WEIGHT	NOTES

WEIGHT LOSS
♡ Tracker ♡

DATE			-/+		WEIGHT	NOTES

WEIGHT LOSS
♡ Tracker ♡

DATE			-/+		WEIGHT	NOTES

WEIGHT LOSS
♡ Tracker ♡

DATE			-/+		WEIGHT	NOTES

WEIGHT LOSS
♡ Tracker ♡

DATE			-/+		WEIGHT	NOTES

WEIGHT LOSS
♡ Tracker ♡

DATE	-/+	WEIGHT	NOTES

WEIGHT LOSS
♡ Tracker ♡

DATE			-/+		WEIGHT	NOTES

WEIGHT LOSS
♡ Tracker ♡

DATE	-/+	WEIGHT	NOTES

WEIGHT LOSS
♡ Tracker ♡

DATE			-/+		WEIGHT	NOTES

WEIGHT LOSS
♡ Tracker ♡

DATE			-/+		WEIGHT	NOTES

WEIGHT LOSS
♡ Tracker ♡

DATE	-/+	WEIGHT	NOTES

WEIGHT LOSS
Tracker

DATE			-/+		WEIGHT	NOTES

WEIGHT LOSS
Tracker

DATE	-/+	WEIGHT	NOTES

WEIGHT LOSS
♡ Tracker ♡

DATE			-/+	WEIGHT	NOTES

WEIGHT LOSS
Tracker

DATE	-/+	WEIGHT	NOTES

WEIGHT LOSS
♡ Tracker ♡

DATE	-/+	WEIGHT	NOTES

WEIGHT LOSS
♡ Tracker ♡

DATE	-/+	WEIGHT	NOTES

WEIGHT LOSS
♡ Tracker ♡

DATE	-/+	WEIGHT	NOTES

WEIGHT LOSS
♡ Tracker ♡

DATE			-/+		WEIGHT	NOTES

WEIGHT LOSS
Tracker

DATE	-/+	WEIGHT	NOTES

WEIGHT LOSS
♡ Tracker ♡

DATE	-/+	WEIGHT	NOTES

WEIGHT LOSS
♡ Tracker ♡

DATE	-/+	WEIGHT	NOTES

WEIGHT LOSS
♡ Tracker ♡

DATE			-/+		WEIGHT	NOTES

WEIGHT LOSS
♡ Tracker ♡

DATE			-/+		WEIGHT	NOTES

WEIGHT LOSS
♡ Tracker ♡

DATE	-/+	WEIGHT	NOTES

WEIGHT LOSS
♡ Tracker ♡

DATE	-/+	WEIGHT	NOTES

WEIGHT LOSS
♡ Tracker ♡

DATE			-/+		WEIGHT	NOTES

WEIGHT LOSS
Tracker

DATE	-/+	WEIGHT	NOTES

WEIGHT LOSS
♡ Tracker ♡

DATE	-/+	WEIGHT	NOTES

WEIGHT LOSS
♡ Tracker ♡

DATE	-/+	WEIGHT	NOTES

WEIGHT LOSS
♡ Tracker ♡

DATE	-/+	WEIGHT	NOTES

WEIGHT LOSS
♡ Tracker ♡

DATE	-/+	WEIGHT	NOTES

WEIGHT LOSS
♡ Tracker ♡

DATE			-/+		WEIGHT	NOTES

WEIGHT LOSS
♡ Tracker ♡

DATE	-/+	WEIGHT	NOTES

WEIGHT LOSS
♡ Tracker ♡

DATE	-/+	WEIGHT	NOTES

WEIGHT LOSS
♡ Tracker ♡

DATE			-/+		WEIGHT	NOTES

WEIGHT LOSS
♡ Tracker ♡

DATE	-/+	WEIGHT	NOTES

WEIGHT LOSS
♡ Tracker ♡

DATE	-/+	WEIGHT	NOTES

WEIGHT LOSS
♡ Tracker ♡

DATE	-/+	WEIGHT	NOTES

WEIGHT LOSS
♡ Tracker ♡

DATE			-/+		WEIGHT	NOTES

WEIGHT LOSS
♡ Tracker ♡

DATE	-/+	WEIGHT	NOTES

WEIGHT LOSS
♡ Tracker ♡

DATE	-/+	WEIGHT	NOTES

WEIGHT LOSS
♡ Tracker ♡

DATE	-/+	WEIGHT	NOTES

WEIGHT LOSS
♡ Tracker ♡

DATE	-/+	WEIGHT	NOTES

WEIGHT LOSS
♡ Tracker ♡

DATE			-/+		WEIGHT	NOTES

WEIGHT LOSS
Tracker

DATE	-/+	WEIGHT	NOTES

Made in the USA
Las Vegas, NV
05 January 2025

15823917R00066